The Secret to Weight Loss For Life

A Beginner's Guide to Losing Weight Quickly, Easily and <u>Permanently</u>!

Ron Kness

Legal Notice:

Disclaimer Notice:

Published by:

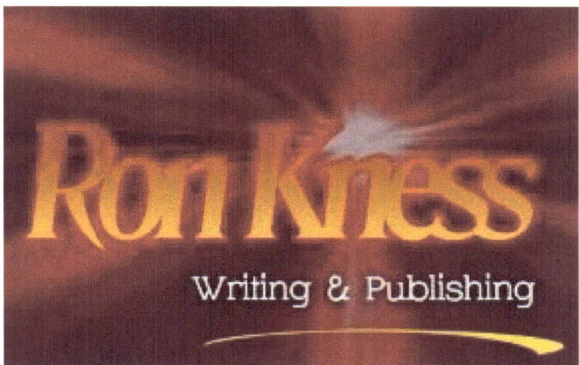

https://ronknesswriting.com

Ron Kness
San Tan Valley, AZ
United States of America

ISBN: 9781080634613

Sneak Peek

Have you ever tried to go on a diet to lose weight, only to find that despite the hunger and frustration, you didn't manage to lose any weight?

Trying to lose weight is a tough and relentless effort. You starve yourself for days hoping to lose a few pounds, only to find yourself no better off than before.

News Flash!!! It doesn't work!

All that works is physical effort. You need discipline, the motivation to change and the "Know How" and then you will get the results you want. It doesn't take anything more than that to get into shape. This guide will give you the "Know How"

If you've been trying to lose weight without any or much success, you may have just stumbled upon something that could finally help you shed those pounds for good - without a single day of starvation!

What Is *Weight Loss For Life* And Who Is It For?

Weight Loss For Life is a brand new guide that will take you by the hand and reveal super simple methods and truths to weight loss that could change your life.

- No matter what situation you are in
- Whether you are Old or Young
- Male or Female
- Come from Poverty or Wealth..

These keys to weight loss success are the same for everyone. They are what's called a universal truth and will work if you have the desire and will to implement them.

Here's Exactly What You Get...

- Assessing your current health situation
- How to do your cardio in a way that burns MORE Fat. And you'll do it in less time!
- The key to understanding Nutrition
- Developing the Right Mindset for Permanent Weight Loss
- Quickly Get Results by Avoiding Common Pitfalls
- 5 Power Foods You Must Have in Your Weight Loss Plan
- And Much, Much More …

Why It's Important to Invest In This Book Right Now…

If you are looking to lose weight quickly, safely and permanently, but don't know where to start, then it's important to not let anything stand in your way from doing it. Don't let a few dollars stop you from learning the secrets that could change your life while also enriching it. Can you put a price on health? And you know that your weight impacts your health.

Get started right away!

And be sure to get our free report by clicking on the image or link below.

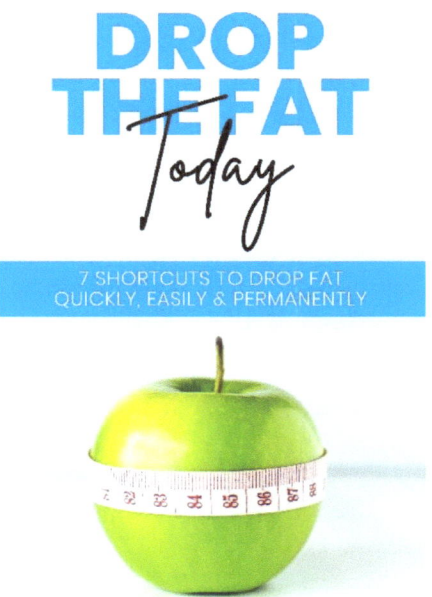

https://secretstoweightlossforlife.s3-us-west-2.amazonaws.com/Lead-Capture-Pages/squeezepage.html

Contents

Introduction

Hello and welcome to our beginners guide on how to lose weight and become healthy quickly, easily and most importantly **permanently**!

On paper, losing weight really is simply a case of burning more calories per day than you eat. In reality, nothing is ever that black and white, and to be truthful, losing weight is one of the hardest processes you will ever endure. And keeping it off is no picnic either!

Lately, health experts and officials have grown increasingly concerned with the obesity epidemic sweeping the nation, and many parts of the developed world.

The number of obese individuals in the world is now at an all-time high. Every single year, it is estimated that more than 2.8 million people lose their lives as a result, either directly or indirectly, of being obese and overweight. Each year, health officials and governments are spending billions on obesity-related healthcare, so something simply must be done before it's too late.

Whereas once upon a time, obesity was prevalent in developed countries with high incomes, recent studies have found that obesity is now growing increasingly common in under-developed countries with poor incomes. This is a very worrying statistic.

While new data is being gathered, we can tell you that back in 2016, the number of overweight individuals living on our planet came in at 1.9 billion. Experts now predict that that number is even higher. Out of these 1.9 billion, a staggering 650 million were obese.

Since the 1970s, obesity levels have tripled, which indicates that somewhere along the line, we're doing things very wrong.

Health Risks Associated with Obesity

Now we're going to take a look at a few major health risks associated with obesity and being overweight.

Type-2 Diabetes – Type-2 Diabetes is very much a condition heavily linked to obesity. The vast majority of people affected with type-2 diabetes are obese or overweight. Losing weight is a great way to manage the disease, and if you do happen to lose weight and lead a healthy lifestyle, you could even potentially rid yourself of the disease entirely.

Heart disease – Heart disease is the number one killer in the world. Each year, more people die from heart disease than from all forms of cancer combined. Being overweight means that your bad cholesterol (LDL) will likely be high, and you will also likely suffer from hypertension (high blood pressure) which can be a precursor for heart disease, as well as other potentially fatal conditions such as a stroke.

Joint issues – People that are overweight often suffer from joint issues such as osteoarthritis. This is because the extra weight that they are carrying is placing additional stress and pressure on their joints. As a matter of fact, for each pound overweight, it puts an additional 5 pounds of stress on your knees. Although the knees often bear the brunt of this weight, back and hip issues are also common with overweight individuals. Losing weight can ease pressure placed on these joints and can therefore improve their overall quality of life.

Fatty liver disease – Individuals who happen to be obese are far more likely to suffer from fatty liver disease. Fatty liver disease is a condition in which the liver literally becomes coated in a restrictive layer of fat. If not addressed, it could potentially be fatal.

Well that's a brief look at the situation we are facing and why it's important to do all we can to increase our health while decreasing obesity

In the first part of the guide we're going to start at the beginning which is our current state of health and the steps to begin a weight loss program correctly.

Are you ready? Let's dive in...

Chapter 1 – Assessing Our Current State Of Health

In life, sadly, nothing worth having seems to come easily, and that unfortunately also seems to apply to good health. If you've ever struggled with your weight in the past, you'll know all too clearly how difficult it is to lose weight.

Losing weight is an arduous, drawn out, stressful, and draining process. To make matters worse, gaining weight seems to be something that many of us can do without even trying. And as you age, losing weight is harder and gaining it becomes even easier!

It can take weeks of diet and exercise to lose a couple of pounds, yet one or two fairly high-calorie meals and that weight can be replaced in the blink of an eye.

Despite weight loss being difficult, it's considered essential for a healthy and prosperous life.

When it comes to our weight however, it's important to monitor our body fat percentages in order to get an accurate reading.

There are a number of different ways of measuring and monitoring body fat levels, with some proving to be more accurate than others. Here's a look at some of the different ways of measuring body fat.

Visit your doctor – This first example is very simple, yet highly recommended. Remember, obesity can literally be fatal and it can lead to all kinds of illnesses, diseases, and ailments.

A visit to your doctor is therefore highly recommended and where any weight loss program should start as they will be able to assess your weight and prescribe you various treatments or refer you to trained specialists such as nutritionists. Your doctor may perform a simple body fat calliper test to measure your body fat, or they may even use the BMI method.

Whatever the case may be, you will have an accurate reading and an assessment from a qualified medical professional that you're good to go. If there are any precautionary measures that you should be aware of, your doctor will inform you about those as well.

BMI – BMI, or Body Mass Index, is arguably the most common method of measuring body fat in the developed world, but it is far from ideal.

Basically, with a BMI test your weight will be measured against your height. If, according to the scales, you are heavier than your optimal weight for somebody your height, you will be classed as overweight, obese, or morbidly obese, depending on how much you are overweight.

Weight, however, does not necessarily equal fat. An average height bodybuilder with a six pack, weighing in at over 230 pounds of solid muscle, would, according to a BMI test, be obese. This is of course not true as that 230 pounds largely comes from muscle, but even so, that's what the BMI test will say.

Weight – If you want to easiest and most primitive method of measuring your body fat, you could invest in a good quality set of weighing scales and weigh yourself.

Weighing scales are far from perfect because they can't differentiate between fat, water, and muscle, but even so, they're great for providing a rough idea of where you're at. If you're looking to lose weight, weighing yourself once a week should give you a good idea of whether your efforts are proving fruitful thus far.

Bio Impedance – Bio Impedance scales are very effective when it comes to measuring body fat because they are able to differentiate between muscle, water, and body fat.

They work by sending out a series of electrical impulses throughout the body, and then measuring the rate in which they return. Electrical currents flow through different materials (fat, muscle, water, etc) at different rates. You simply stand on the specially designed scales and you'll find that the results are with you in a matter of seconds.

Take "Progress" Photo's - This is a very important step and with just about everyone having a smartphone, it just takes seconds to snap a photo of your body. Take one photo with you facing forward and one photo of your side profile... similar to what you see in the weight loss magazines.

Photos are probably the best indicator of how far you've come in your weight loss journey. A general rule of thumb is that in the first 30 days, you may see your weight drop a little and you'll notice the difference, but your family and friends probably won't.

By the 60th day, there'll definitely be a visible difference and your family members will start to take notice that you are getting slimmer.

By the 90th day, just about everyone who knows you will have to admit that you've shed the pounds and you look fitter, healthier and have a certain glow about you.

The question now is... Will you reach day 90? The second question is ... will you keep off the weight?

The photos that you take once every 3 weeks or monthly will keep you going. If you rely on the weight that you see on a scale, you may probably give up like thousands of people who do.

There's a reason for this. The scale does not show how much fat you've lost and how much muscle you've gained. People who start training after a long period of being sedentary can gain lean muscle quite quickly. The body is craving muscle and grabs the chance to build some when you're eating and training right.

For example, if you lose 7 pounds of fat but gain 3 pounds of muscle at the end of a month, the scale will reflect a drop of only 4 pounds. This can be very discouraging to many people because they were expecting better results.

What they don't realize is that muscle is denser than fat. An equal amount of muscle weighs more than the same amount of fat. So, by losing 7 pounds of fat, there will be a significant difference in your appearance.

Your jawline may become more pronounced. Your thighs may have stopped rubbing against each other when you walk and your arms may be much more toned.

But you can't see any of these results on a scale. That is exactly why you should take photos every now and then. When you compare your before and after photos, you'll be amazed at how much change there is... and these positive changes will spur you to do better and give more. You'll stay the course and be motivated to reach your weight loss goal. Keep in mind, your scale is only one tool of many that you should be using to track your weight loss.

This is about all you need to do to assess your current situation. In the next part, we'll look at the most crucial factor that determines if you'll lose weight successfully or join the majority of people who never succeed at it and battle with their weight all their lives...setting goals & sticking to them!

Chapter 2 – Setting Productive Weight Loss Goals and Motivational Techniques

As you know, obesity can potentially be fatal, which is why it's so important for us to get our weight under control as quickly as we possibly can.

The sooner we act, the longer we will hopefully live. If you're serious about losing weight, it's vital that you stick with the plan for the long-haul.

There are no shortcuts when it comes to losing weight, nor are there any quick fixes. If you're serious about losing weight, it's important to set yourself goals. Goal setting however, is easier said than done. To stick to your goals, you need to ensure that you are motivated and driven.

"Weight loss is not a physical challenge. It's a mental one."

Before you even set any weight loss goals it's time for a reality check. Here are a few things you need to know and be aware of:

- Losing 1 or 2 pounds of fat a week is normal and considered a healthy loss rate.
- The more overweight you are, the more fat you will lose in the initial stages. As you progress, your weight loss results will start tapering down.
- There may be a week or two when the numbers on the scale just don't change… or might even go up a pound.
- Your caloric deficit is the most important factor.
- It takes time to lose weight.

Now that we've got that out of the way, here's a look at how to set goals and stay motivated.

Set realistic goals – When losing weight, the temptation is always there to set yourself an outrageous weight loss goal in a bid to help keep yourself driven and focussed. At first this technique may prove beneficial, but as time goes by and reality sets in, you'll begin to realise that, actually, the goals you set are not really viable.

Losing 3 pounds in a week for example, is quite tough, but it is realistic. Setting a goal of losing 10 pounds in a week though, is not realistic or practical. If for example, you lost 4 pounds that week, ordinarily that would be an extraordinary loss. Because you set a goal of 10, as you would be 6 pounds light, you'd view it as a failure.

This would then result in you adopting much more of a negative mindset. When you set weight loss goals, they must always be realistic and attainable. For more information on the role of mindset in regard to losing weight get my new book *The Psychology Behind Weight Loss.*

Visualise — When we attempt to lose weight and get in shape, we will experience emotional highs and lows. Some days we'll find ourselves full of energy and motivation, and ready to tackle whatever the day throws at us. Other days however, we find ourselves tired, unmotivated, and questioning why we're even bothering.

When you feel like this, visualise your goals and targets and remember why you're losing weight in the first place. Visualise yourself leaner, fitter, healthier, and happier and focus on how much better you will look and feel.

Make small goals and meet them - Once you start cleaning up your diet and eating wholesome, nutritious food, your goal can be to slowly eliminate the detrimental foods over time. As far as your training regimen goes, your goal may be to get to the gym 3 or 4 times a week or walk daily. It doesn't have to be huge goals. Aim for ones that you can manage and each week, make small improvements. Small improvements over time add up to be big changes.

While we've covered setting goals & motivation, the real work is about to begin. In the next chapter we'll look at nutrition and the fundamentals of a healthy diet.

Chapter 3 – Nutritional Overview – The Fundamentals of a Healthy Diet

As you know, health is wealth, and if you want to lose weight to get fit and healthy, you need to begin by addressing your diet.

When we think of diets, we think of miniscule portions, salad, vegetables, and other bland and tasteless foods that maybe good for us, but are hardly inspiring when it comes to taste.

In truth, the entire concept behind a healthy diet is extremely complex as there is a lot to get your head around. While we won't be going into too much technical detail when looking at diet and nutrition, we will be providing a basic nutritional overview and will be looking at some of the basic fundamentals associated with a healthy diet.

Hydration – First and foremost, it doesn't matter which diet and nutritional plan you intend on following, adequate hydration is absolutely essential. The human body is made up of close to 80% water.

We need water for our cells to function properly, we need water to digest our food, we need water to convert calories into energy, we need water for our organs to function properly, and we need water to simply feel healthy and productive. Water helps speed up the metabolism and promotes athletic performance, making adequate hydration perfect for people trying to lose weight.

As well as that, water is also very beneficial for the brain. Experts recommend that we consume around 8 glasses of water each day. Avoid sugary drinks, as well as sugar-free drinks which are loaded with chemicals, and instead get your hydration from fresh mineral or filtered water. If you get tired of drinking just plain water, make your own infused water.

Macros – Macros, or macronutrients if we're being technical, are made up of: fats, proteins, and carbohydrates. Basically, these are your three macronutrients. It is worth noting roughly how many calories the different types of macronutrients contain.

- Carbohydrates - 4 calories per gram
- Proteins - 4 calories per gram

- Fats - 9 calories per gram

Notice that fat has over twice the calories as the other two macronutrients, but we need a healthy balance of all three macros as they perform different functions and processes within the body.

Protein for example, is used to help repair and rebuild damaged muscle tissue. It's also vital for cellular health and function. Carbohydrates are typically used by the body as a key source of energy, whereas fats are used to regulate your hormones, boost the metabolism, promote healthy organs, and much more besides.

When trying to lose weight, your macronutrient ratios should be at 50% protein, 35% carbs and 15% fat.

Micronutrients – Micronutrients are another group of essential food groups needed by the body in order for it to function at its best. Micronutrients generally consist of vitamins and minerals. These all play incredibly important roles in the body and are vital for optimal health and well-being.

We need vitamins for a healthy immune system, for wound healing, for organ function, for energy production, for hormone regulation, and much more besides.

Minerals are equally as important as each one offers unique benefits and advantages to the body. Minerals such as calcium for example, are important for strong and healthy bones. Iron is a mineral essential for the blood as it plays a key role in the production haemoglobin.

Calories – Calories are basically units of energy. The human body needs energy for a whole variety of different reasons. We get our energy from food and drink. The amount of energy found in each food and drinks item is measured in calories.

To maintain itself in its current state, the body needs a certain number of calories. This number varies from person to person. If we consume more calories than the body needs for maintenance, we create a caloric surplus.

Rather than letting these calories go to waste, the body instead converts them into fat and stores them to be used at a later date. During our caveman days, this biologic process was important because they never knew where their next meal was coming and the additional fat carried them through during the lean times to prevent starvation. While that is no longer a problem for most of us, the process is still there. We can't change the process, but we can use it to our advantage. How?

By not consuming enough calories needed for maintenance, we create a caloric deficit and the body taps into its fat reserves to make up the difference. This is a very simple explanation of how a caloric deficit promotes weight loss.

Are You Carb Sensitive?

This is a HUGE problem that is the underlying cause for why fat people keep getting fatter… and the rate of weight gain is accelerated.

Some people are highly carb sensitive. When they consume even a little bit of carbs, they gain weight fast. This is due to insulin insensitivity. You're probably wondering what causes this. The answer is quite simple.

Let's assume you drink a can of sugary soda. The sugar in the soda will spike your blood sugar levels. Your body will release insulin to prevent your blood sugar level from getting too high (hyperglycemia).

Now if you were to drink 3 cans of soda a day, your body will keep releasing insulin to cope with these elevated sugar levels. Over time, your body will get desensitized to the insulin and your pancreas will have to keep releasing more insulin just to cope with the same amount of sugar.

When this happens, the excess insulin will be shuttled off to the body's fat stores through a chain of processes within the body. This will explain why overweight people often complain that they eat 1 slice of cake and gain 4 pounds.

While this is a bit of an exaggeration, you do get the point. A long time of consuming junk food and processed foods has affected their body's internal system.

Another very nasty consequence of insulin insensitivity is that it sets the stage for type 2 diabetes which is the leading cause of kidney failure, blindness and amputations. This is one of the worst diseases out there... and it all starts from a poor diet.

So what do I do if I'm insulin insensitive?

There are a few ways to reduce insulin insensitivity. Thousands of people will see rapid weight loss if they 'reset' their body's insulin sensitivity.

This is one of the biggest weight loss hurdles that most people aren't even aware of. Fix your insulin insensitivity and it will become much easier to shed the stubborn pounds. Here are a few methods.

- Reduce your intake of all sugary and refined foods till you can eliminate them completely.
- Consume more foods which contain turmeric/ginger/garlic.
- Get enough sleep daily. This is very important. If you get insufficient sleep, consume some cinnamon. This will help attenuate the effects of the insulin resistance that arises from insufficient sleep.
- Lift weights.
- Run three times a week in a fasted state.
- Drink unsweetened green tea regularly. The gallic acid in the tea will improve your insulin sensitivity.
- Consume leafy greens and food rich in magnesium.
- Reduce or totally stop your intake of refined carbs like white rice, white bread, pasta, etc.

Just by following these steps, you'd have done the single biggest thing to help yourself progress faster in your weight loss journey. Get started on it today... and move on to the next chapter!

Chapter 4 – Top 5 Power Foods You Need In Your Diet For Weight Loss

To some people, the thought of eating food to lose weight is preposterous. Surely, when it comes to losing weight the less food you eat, the better? In reality however, the exact opposite is true.

To lose weight, we need to make sure that we've eaten enough of the right foods to provide our metabolisms with the energy needed to function. Some foods, however, are even more beneficial for shedding the pounds than others.

Here's a look at the top 5 power foods for weight loss.

Broccoli – Broccoli is a superfood which is considered one of the healthiest in the world. If you're looking to lose weight, broccoli is ideal.

To begin with, broccoli is naturally low in calories and is virtually fat-free. As well as that, broccoli is also rich in fiber, which is your secret weapon in the battle against the bulge. Fiber helps to promote satiety and helps to keep you feeling full for longer. If you feel full, you'll be less likely to overeat.

Salmon – Salmon is an oily fish that is renowned for its health benefits. Salmon is a rich source of protein which is very useful for burning fat. Protein is thermogenic, which means that it raises your core body temperature as it is broken down.

This in turn means that your body burns off more calories just to digest the food and break it down. The weight loss benefits here are apparent. As an added bonus, salmon is also rich in omega-3 fatty acids and essential minerals.

Chicken breast – If you look at any healthy eating plan containing meat, you'll find that the primary protein source is usually chicken breast.

For losing weight, chicken breast is ideal. Chicken breast is virtually fat-free when skinless, and is naturally low in calories.

It's also a great source of protein, which increases your metabolism as it is digested and broken down. Not only that, but as protein takes longer to digest and be broken down, it also stays in your stomach for longer so you feel full for longer, which means you are less likely to snack on unhealthy foods between meals..

Avocados – Avocados are naturally rich in fats and are high in calories. Because of this, people often avoid them when trying to lose weight. This is a mistake. You see, avocados are rich in healthy fats such as oleic acid, which has been found to ramp up the metabolism and fight inflammation.

Inflammation is heavily linked with obesity. Avocados are also a great source of fiber. This, combined with their high-calorie content, makes them perfect for keeping you feeling full for longer.

Coconut oil – Coconut oil is roughly 99% saturated fat. The saturated fat found in coconut oil however, is incredibly good for you.

The fats found in coconut oil are MCTs, or Medium Chain Triglycerides. Because of their triglyceride chain length, when consumed, these fats are used as a near-instant source of energy.

The body is able to use the fat for fuel quicker, so you don't store the fats for use at a later date. This increase in energy means that your metabolism increases, and you will therefore burn more calories. Hooray for coconuts.

Well these are just a few power foods everyone should look at including into a healthy and balanced diet. In the next part we will look at some of the most popular diets going around and whether they should be implemented or thrown in the trash bin.

Chapter 5 – Popular Diets and Fad Diets – Which Should You Choose?

If you decide that you need to lose weight, what's the first plan of action that springs to mind? For the vast majority of us, it's to go on a diet.

The word 'diet' is actually very broad because there are literally hundreds of different diet plans out there for people to choose from.

Needless to say, some are incredibly effective, whereas others, not so much. Some diets have proven to be effective and have been backed up by science and medical research. Others, however, are nothing more than passing fads, and can potentially be dangerous.

Keep in mind most diets are meant for short-term loss. They are fine if you are wanting to shed a few pounds in preparation for some event, like a high school reunion or a wedding for example. But they were never meant to be long-term.

And because most diets restrict or eliminate one or more food groups, the body eventually craves the food it is no longer getting and will raise its ugly head in the form of cravings. Regardless of your willpower cravings will win out every time. When that happens, you go back to your old way of eating, put in the weight you lost (and more in most cases) and choose a different diet to go on to lose the weight you gained back. Sound familiar? The reality is yo-yo dieting is harder on the body than being a few pounds overweight and staying there. A much better approach to "dieting" is choosing a healthy eating plan that you can live on for life as part of an overall healthy lifestyle. No more yo-yo dieting!

Here are some popular diets to consider, and some fads to steer well clear of.

Popular diets

We'll start off on a high by looking at popular diets that have enjoyed a lot of success and have been found to be effective. If you're looking to lose weight and improve your health in the process, you may wish to consider the following:

The paleo diet – The paleo diet is sometimes known as the caveman diet. It has the word 'diet' in it, but in truth it is more of a lifestyle change.

The basic premise is that followers of the diet eat foods similar to what cavemen used to eat hundreds of thousands of years ago. The diet isn't as much about losing weight, as it is about eating natural, non-processed food the way evolution intended. A bonus however, is that you will lose weight.

Keto – Ketogenic diets are hugely popular nowadays. Keto diets are low carb, moderate protein, high fat diets that cause your body to enter ketosis. When this occurs, you produce ketones via fat cells, which are then used for energy. By default, you are technically using fat for energy, rather than carbohydrates.

5:2 diet – The 5:2 diet is a form of intermittent fasting. Basically, on this diet you will eat normal foods for 5 days of the week, and for 2 days you'll consume just 500 calories. If you stick to the diet and DO NOT binge on your normal eating days, you can potentially lose a lot of weight.

Fad diets to avoid

Now we'll look at some fad diets to avoid if you value your health:

Cabbage soup diet – The cabbage soup diet is as disgusting as it sounds. With this diet, the idea is that you primarily consume low-calorie cabbage soup every day, and that you consume around 800 calories on average.

You will lose weight, but it is not sustainable. Not only that, but the longer the cabbage is cooked, the more nutrients it loses.

Raw food diet – As the name implies, this is a diet in which you only really consume foods in their raw form. Does that mean you should eat raw meat? No.

The raw food diet only permits foods which can safely be consumed raw, I.E fruits, nuts, and veggies. Eating most vegetables raw is a great way of getting more nutrients, but the diet isn't sustainable.

Cotton ball diet – This diet should be banished from the face of the earth forever. The cotton ball diet is a diet in which people literally soak cotton wool balls in fresh juices or green tea, and then swallow them.

Why? The "logic" behind swallowing cotton balls is that they swell up in your stomach and take longer to digest, so you feel full for longer. The fuller you feel, the less you eat. This diet is very dangerous and could kill you. Don't do it – ever!

So which is the best one for you?

There is no right or wrong answer here because this book is not about teaching you to live your entire life on any one diet. While you may choose one to help you lose weight in the short-term, ideally, the best thing that you can do is change your eating habits for the better.

A lot of diets have stringent rules and try to exclude certain foods that are deemed anathema to the diet. For example, the paleo diet doesn't allow you to consume artificial ingredients, grains and dairy.

This can be a nightmarish diet for people who love having the occasional cake and ice-cream. While there are paleo alternatives, they just don't quite cut it. Because of this, adhering to such strict diets can be a turn off for many people.

The key to succeeding with weight loss and keeping off the excess pounds is moderation. Life is too short for you to avoid the foods you love completely. Approach your eating from a mindful aspect. This book can help you understand this concept.

What you need to do is replace most of your unhealthy food choices with healthier ones… and occasionally indulge - on a limited and infrequent basis - in the foods you love. Healthy eating should be a lifestyle choice and not because you're forcing yourself to be on a diet.

Include lots of vegetables in your diet. Have fruit for snacks. Replace sodas with water or unsweetened green tea. Cut down your intake of processed foods.

Follow the right macronutrient combinations. If your diet consisted mainly of single ingredient foods, you'd be just fine. A broccoli is a single ingredient food. Canned vegetable soup is not.

Like the late fitness guru Jack LaLanne once said, *"If man made it, don't eat it."*

As long as you are on track most of the time, it's fine to indulge in the occasional treat. Treating yourself to a food you love in moderation once every 4 or 5 days is just fine. In fact, it will give you a mental break and make you happier.

Drink lots of water because water helps in the fat loss process. Drink a glass of water before each meal. This will not only make you fuller and prevent you from overeating, but it'll also keep you hydrated for your workouts.

Have a teaspoon of cumin seeds every day. This will help you lose 3 times more fat. It's such a simple practice but so powerful.

Consume one tablespoon of cold pressed coconut oil daily. This will further help in your weight loss progress. As counter-intuitive as it may seem, you must consume good fat in order to lose fat. When your body realizes that it has a steady supply of fat coming in, it will be much more ready to burn off its fat stores. This is the basic premise behind the keto diet.

Coconut oil received a bad reputation in the past. However, recent studies have shown that it is one of the best foods around and prevents a myriad of health issues.

Chapter 6 – Weight Loss Nutrition Shopping Tips

When you make a conscious effort to lose weight and take back your health, you need to ensure that you're doing everything in your power to consume the right foods at the right times.

This is where it pays dividends to know what you're doing when you're out browsing the grocery store for healthy foods and drinks.

To help make your shopping trips for healthy food that little bit easier, we're going to share a series of healthy shopping tips with you right now. And because we're so generous and helpful, we're also going to share a sample healthy meal plan for the day with you, so you have a better idea of the types of things you should be eating to lose weight.

Weight loss nutrition shopping tips

To get things started, here's a look at some useful shopping tips for when you're looking to stock up on healthy, weight loss friendly foods and drinks.

Never go shopping hungry — If there's just one piece of advice to take heed of, let it be this: Never go food shopping for healthy produce when you're hungry.

When you're hungry, you won't be thinking clearly, you'll be craving something quick, easy, and tasty, and you'll be surrounded by unhealthy junk food that you'll find hard to resist. If you've already eaten a healthy meal however, you'll be full, and you won't be interested in the junk food at all.

Don't buy food labelled as 'low fat' — Although you're looking to lose weight, you should still avoid food labelled as being 'low fat' at all costs. This is because low-fat alternatives to everyday food items often contain ingredients that are far worse.

Normally they'll be packed full of artificial flavorings, chemicals, sweeteners, and preservatives which do the body no good at all. Sure, they may be low in fat and calories, but they're still very unhealthy.

Read the packaging and ingredients – If you're unsure about whether or not something is healthy, read the packaging and take a look at the list of ingredients found inside.

If there are dozens upon dozens of ingredients, including chemicals that you can't pronounce, it's not healthy and it should be ignored. Look for foods and products containing natural ingredients.

Don't fear frozen vegetables – There's a misconception in the world of dieting, that frozen vegetables are unhealthy. In reality, most frozen veggies are simply coated with fresh water and frozen at source, making them very fresh. Some fruit and veg you see on grocery shelves, could have been standing for weeks and may not be as fresh as you'd like. The fresher the produce, the higher the nutrient count.

Sample healthy menu
- Breakfast
  - Slice of wholegrain toast
  - Half a smashed avocado
  - 1 poached egg
  - 1 serving of wilted spinach
- Snack
  - 1 apple
- Lunch
  - 1 homemade chicken and Mediterranean vegetable salad with vinaigrette dressing
- Snack
  - 1 yogurt
  - 1 handful of mixed berries
- Dinner
  - 1 baked cod fillet
  - 1 serving of fresh asparagus
  - 1 baked sweet potato
- Snack
  - 1 serving of cottage cheese
  - 1 handful of mixed nuts

Now that we've learned a few shopping tips while on a weight loss plan, the next thing we will look at is adding exercise into the mix.

Keep in mind that losing weight is 80% nutrition and 20% exercise. But exercising has other benefits besides burning additional calories as we will see.

Chapter 7 - Introducing Exercise into a Weight Loss Regime

If you were to ask any health expert what the two basic fundamentals of weight loss were, they'd tell you diet and exercise.

Exercise is extremely misunderstood when it comes to losing weight, yet when it is performed correctly, it can really speed up the process and improve your health to no end.

But just what is it about exercise that makes it so beneficial? Sure, it's easy to sit here and tell you that exercise is healthy, but why is it healthy? What does exercise do for you that makes it healthy, and how can you introduce an exercise and fitness routine into a weight loss regime?

Let's find out, shall we?

Health benefits of exercise

To begin with, we're going to start by looking at some of the main health benefits of exercise. These include, but are not limited to:

Weight loss – Yes, we're as shocked as you are, but yes, it turns out that exercise does in fact help you to lose weight. Who knew, right?

When we exercise and exert ourselves physically, our bodies of course need energy to perform the various activities we're performing. This energy comes from calories we consume as well as those found in stored body fat. The more physically active we are, the more calories we burn and the more weight we will lose.

Cardiovascular health – One of the biggest risks of obesity is heart disease. Heart disease is the number one killer in the world, and what's even more frustrating is the fact that it can be avoided by following a healthy diet and lifestyle.

Exercise is beneficial for the heart and cardiovascular system as it reduces blood pressure, it lowers LDL cholesterol, it improves circulation, and it strengthens the heart, making it more effective.

Improved mental health — Have you ever noticed how, after exercising you feel fantastic? You're full of energy, you're in a great mood, you feel alert, and you just feel happier and more content with life.

Exercise promotes the production and secretion of endorphins and other happy chemicals that improve your mood and improve your mental health. Exercise can potentially be a fantastic natural treatment for mental health issues such as stress, anxiety, and depression.

Exercise boosts your energy levels — If you ever find yourself feeling tired, lethargic, and fatigued, exercise is perfect. One would think it would have the opposite effect — making you more tired, but because of the "feel good" hormones released it is almost a euphoric effect.

Studies have found that regular exercise can increase a person's energy levels significantly. Exercise boosts the metabolism, which in turn generates more energy for you, while burning off more calories in the process.

Should you work out at a gym or at home?

People often wonder whether it's more effective to train at a gym, or to simply exercise at home. Here's a look at some pros and cons of each.

Gym pros:

- More equipment
- Great atmosphere
- Plenty of variety
- Access to personal trainers and experts

Gym cons:

- Travel
- Price
- Can get busy at times

Exercise at home pros:

- Save time
- No large crowds
- Save money
- Do your own thing
- Listen to your own music

Exercise at home cons:

- Potential lack of space
- Lack of equipment
- Hard to get motivated sometimes
- Can get boring

Well that's a brief overview for and against training at home or at a gym. The main takeaway should be to stay focused on your weight loss goals we set and exercise regularly. You must be stronger than your excuses and it's when you feel like skipping your training the most that you absolutely must get up and do that 5 minutes. This will boost your self-esteem and you'll develop the mindset of a winner.

And you're a winner, aren't you? Of course you are! You're still reading this... and you should carry on reading the next chapter.

Chapter 8 – Cardio Training - HIIT or Steady State?

Exercise is a critical component of any weight loss regime and when we think of exercise for weight loss, we think of cardio.

Cardiovascular exercise is incredibly beneficial for the heart. In fact, the word 'cardio' is derived from the Ancient Greek word 'Kardia' which literally meant 'heart'.

Lately, more and more people have been performing HIIT as part of their cardio workouts, but is HIIT more beneficial than steady state? That's what we're going to attempt to find out right now.

What is HIIT?

HIIT, or High Intensity Interval Training, is a form of training in which individuals alternate between periods of slow and steady exercise and fast-paced high intensity exercise.
The individual performing the workout will perform a short burst of slow and steady exercise, following by high intensity fast-paced bursts of energy for a number of different rounds.

A typical HIIT workout is over in far less time than a steady state cardio workout, as it typically lasts just 15 – 30 minutes on average.

Benefits of HIIT

Saves time – HIIT workouts are over in no more than 30 minutes on average. In fact, the average workout lasts just 20 minutes. During this time, you can burn off as many calories as you would with a one-hour steady state cardio session.

Burns calories – Just because HIIT workouts are over quickly that doesn't mean that they aren't effective. HIIT workouts are incredibly physically demanding and in just 20 minutes you can potentially burn off more than 400 calories.

Not only that, but because it is so physically demanding, your metabolism increases after the exercise is complete and you burn off more calories than usual, even while in a rested state. This is known as the afterburn effect.

Keeps things interesting — We wouldn't exactly call HIIT workouts fun, unless you're a sadist, but we would say that they keep things interesting.

A typical steady state cardio workout performed on a treadmill can be boring. You're literally going at the same pace, looking at the same view for close to an hour. With HIIT, you're constantly changing the workout, so things stay fresh and exciting.

Simple Sample HIIT workout

After warming up, get onto a treadmill, set it to a very slow pace, and walk for 60 seconds. Now, increase the speed and sprint as fast as you can for 40 seconds.

Turn the speed to low, walk for 60 seconds, and repeat for as many rounds as you can fit in in the space of 20 minutes.

Other HIIT workouts include a circuit of several different exercises where you do the exercise for a set time as hard as you can, rest for twice that amount of time, move onto the next exercise and repeat the process. Repeat the circuit as many times as you can in 20 minutes.

What is steady state cardio?

Steady state cardio is basically a continuous cardio-based workout performed at a moderate speed, for a long duration of time. Typically, a steady state cardio workout will last 45 – 60 minutes.

Benefits of steady state cardio

Easier – Steady state cardio is much easier than HIIT, making it ideal for beginners .

Better on the joints – Walking at a steady pace on a treadmill, or outdoors, is much easier on the joints than sprinting on a hard surface.

Burns calories – Steady state cardio is still cardio, and it is therefore great for people looking to lose weight.

Sample steady state cardio workout

After stretching and warming up, either go for a long walk outdoors, or jump on a treadmill and walk at a steady pace for around 45 – 60 minutes. It's that simple.

Well that's an overview of cardio training and the difference between high intensity intervals and steady state cardio. In the next part we will look at ramping up your exercise efforts and add resistance training into your weight loss plan.

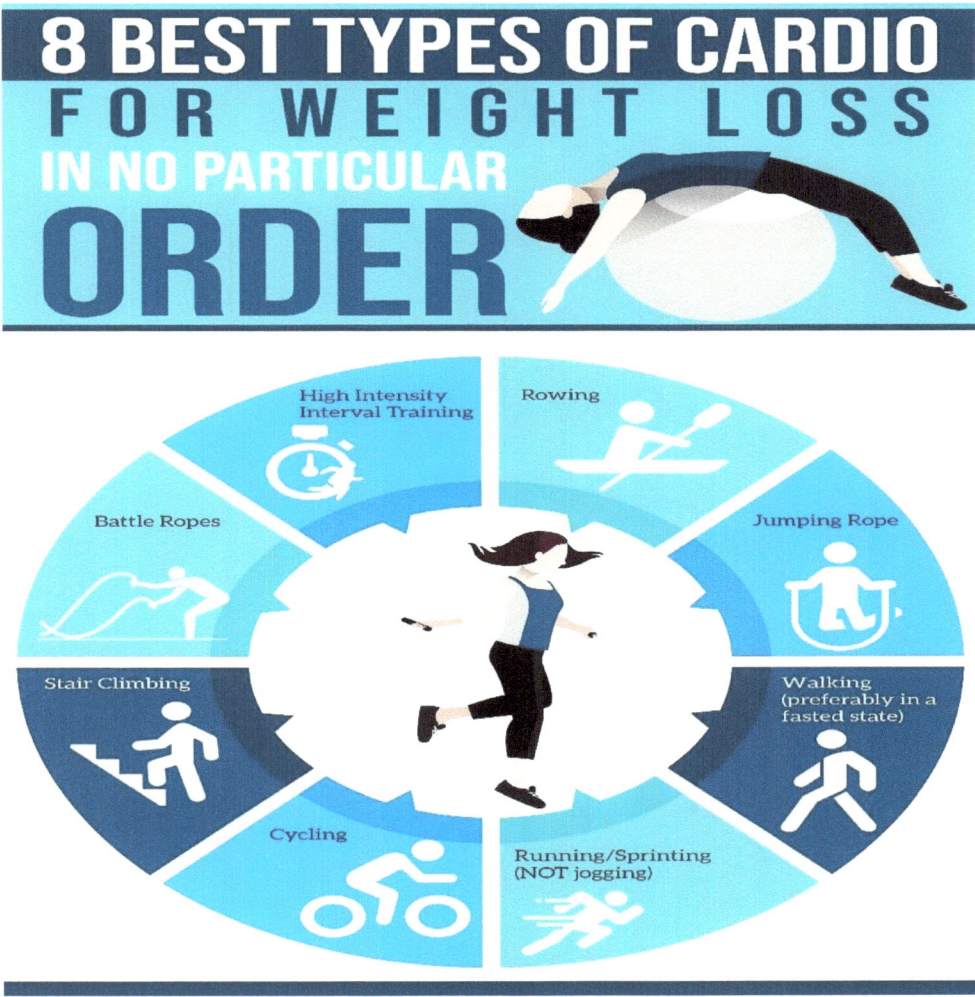

Chapter 9 – The Importance of Resistance Training

Exercise is hugely beneficial to us for a whole variety of different reasons. When it comes to weight loss however, people generally tend to think of cardio which we covered in the last chapter.

While cardiovascular exercise is indeed very effective for burning fat, we shouldn't overlook the importance of resistance training. Resistance training with weights is so beneficial, yet many of us overlook it for fear of getting "too big" and "too muscular".

Here's a look at why resistance training is so beneficial for our health and well-being in general.

Builds muscle — This is, ironically, the one aspect of resistance training that puts some people off. For some people, being big and muscular is very appealing, but for others, not so much.

The reality is that weight and resistance training will build lean muscle if you're consistent, but if you're worried about looking like an enormous 280-pound bodybuilder then please don't as that simply won't happen.

What will likely happen however, is you will gain a few pounds of lean muscle which will help you to look better, burn more calories than before and also help protect you from injury.

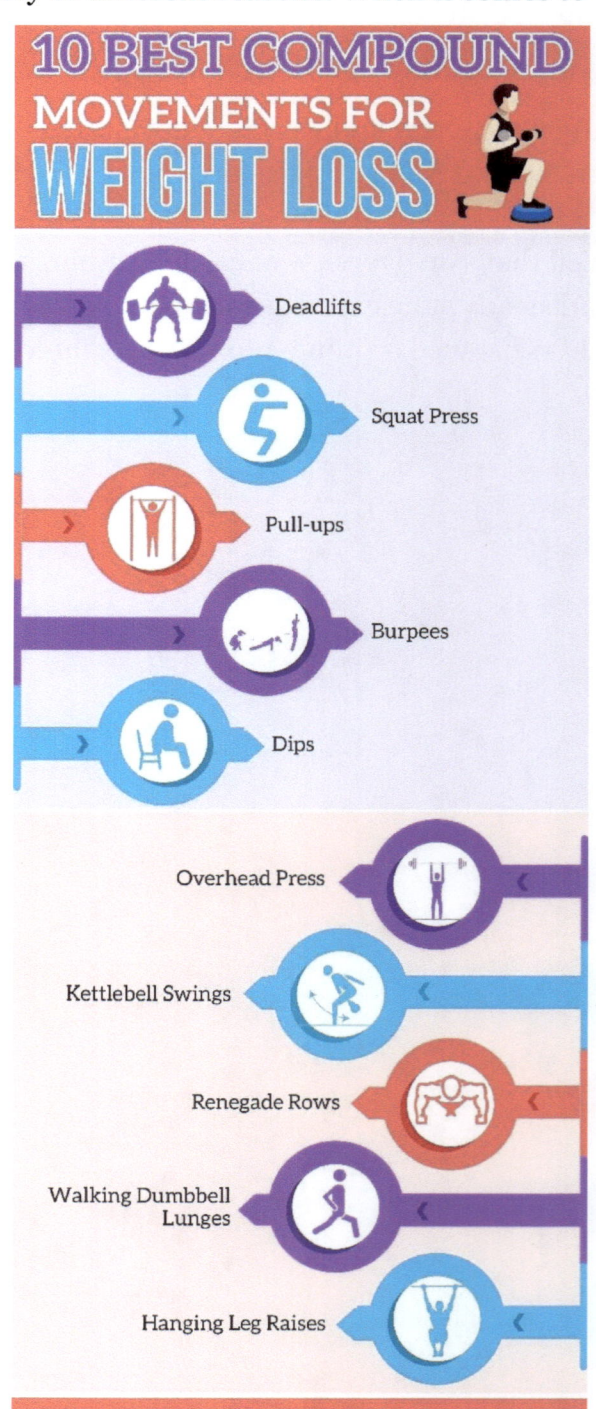

Burns fat — People still seem to be amazed by the fact that resistance training does in fact help promote fat loss.

If you lift weights and train like a bodybuilder, you will build muscle which could cause you to gain weight. The weight you gain is muscle, and this is what people struggle to realise.

Resistance training is a form of exercise that promotes fat loss. You're still burning calories when you exert yourself. Not only that, but as you increase your lean muscle mass your metabolism increases so you burn off even more calories than usual. If you want to burn fat and get leaner, resistance training is no only great … it is a must!

Great for the bones — As we grow older, our bone health often begins to deteriorate. This is where resistance training is so useful.

Resistance training has been found to help strengthen the bones and protect them from age-related damage as we grow older. Resistance training can help to strengthen the bones and prevent conditions such as: osteoarthritis and osteoporosis.

Reduced risk of injury — When you engage in any form of physical exercise or exertion, there's always a risk of injury. Resistance training, however, has been found to help reduce the likelihood of you suffering an injury.

Resistance training helps to build up the muscles and strengthen the bones, muscles, and joints, offering them an element of protection. Put simply, a small and frail body is far more susceptible to injury than a lean and muscular body.

Bodyweight training VS Free weights

If you prefer not to train with weights and keep things 'natural' there are a ton of bodyweight training exercises that are just as challenging. In fact, certain bodyweight exercises are so difficult that even people who have been training with free weights for years can't do them.

Planche pushups, front levers, V-sits, pistol squats, etc. are some of the most difficult bodyweight exercises in existence. If you can do them, you can rest assured that you will be strong and lean.

There are hundreds of bodyweight exercises and variations that will keep you busy for a long time. By the time you master them, you'd have reached your weight loss goal and be hard as nails.

It's next to impossible to get bulky with bodyweight training. So, if that's a concern of yours, bodyweight training has your name written all over it.

To see a variety of bodyweight exercises, all you need to do is go on YouTube and search for these exercises and try them out. Always be safe and approach the training in a sensible manner.

It would be good to mix bodyweight training with free weights. Neither is better than the other. The goal here is to work your muscles and it doesn't matter which method you choose as long as you get there.

Many people feel intimidated going to a gym and would prefer to train at home. Others find it a hassle and some even balk at the cost of the gym memberships. Some folks are even put off at having to use machines that have other people's sweat on them.

The good news is that your muscles do not care where you work out. So you can either get free weights and train at home or just do bodyweight training in the privacy of your own home. Just make sure resistance training is part of your workout regimen.

When you lift heavy weights, your body exerts and the muscles get a hard workout. When you're trying to lose weight, your resistance training should mostly comprise of full-body workouts.

Unlike bodybuilders who train one or two body parts a day, you should be doing several different exercises that target muscles all over the body.

A sample workout would be like the one below.

Sample bodyweight circuit – Run through these exercises 2 or 3 times per workout:

- Deadlifts – 45 seconds followed by 15 seconds rest
- Push-ups – 45 seconds followed by 15 seconds rest
- Squats - 45 seconds followed by 15 seconds rest

- Hanging leg raises - 45 seconds followed by 15 seconds rest
- Burpees - 45 seconds followed by 15 seconds rest
- Lunges - 45 seconds followed by 15 seconds rest

By doing the workout above, not only would you have targeted several different muscles in the body but the minimal rest would have made the resistance training workout take on a cardio nature.

So, you'll be toning your muscles and improving your stamina at the same time. You'll be killing two birds with one stone. Not only that, but the workout will be exhausting and put you in calorie burning mode for several hours after your training session is over.

This will help you burn more calories overall and lose weight faster than you ever expected. However, the effects of overtraining can be as bad as not training at all. In the next part, we look at getting proper rest and recovery - an essential part of a weight loss plan.

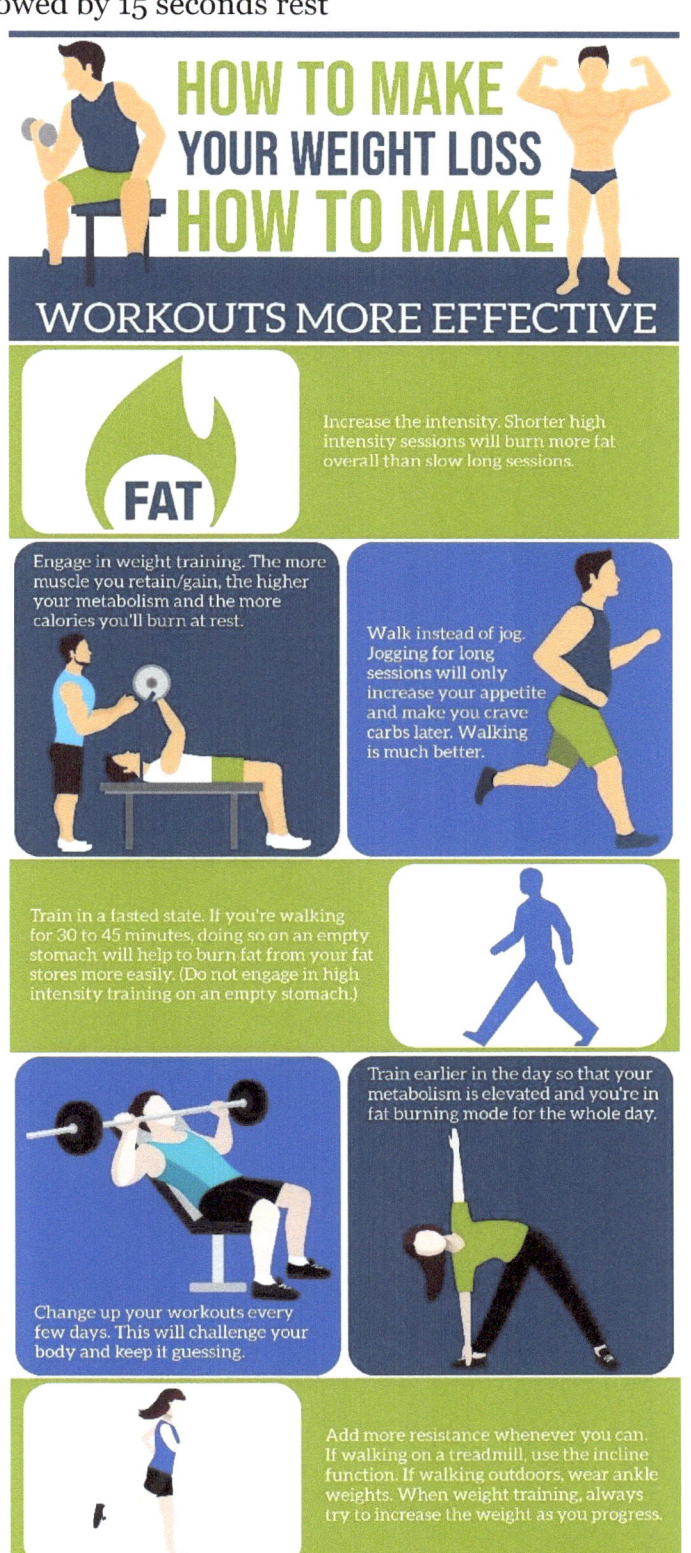

Chapter 10 - Rest and Recovery – The Importance of Rest Days

We know that to burn calories and lose weight, you need to really be pushing yourself in the gym while training. It's no use going to the gym and simply going through the motions; to get the most from your training, you need to get serious about doing it.

However, a crucial, and often overlooked element of any weight loss training regime, is rest and recovery. Rest days are just as important as training days, in fact, some would argue that they're more important.

Here's a look at why rest and recovery days are so important.

Aids in Recovery – After you finish a gruelling workout, you'll probably have noticed how your body aches and you feel sore. This is because you've literally damaged your muscles through training. For the muscles to repair themselves, you need to rest. When we rest, our bodies repair the damage we caused when training, and they rebuild the muscles even bigger and stronger than they used to be. If you don't get enough rest, your muscles won't rebuild and you won't gain lean muscle mass.

Prevents overtraining – Contrary to popular belief, there is such a thing as overtraining, and if you push yourself too hard, too frequently, and don't get in rest days, you do indeed run the risk of overtraining. Overtraining means that you are literally doing too much exercise and are not allowing your body to catch up and recover.

Overtraining can result in muscle wastage, it can suppress the metabolism, it will leave you feeling tired, sore, and lethargic, and it can potentially result in you gaining weight. When it comes to working out, rest days are just important as training days.

Prevents injury – When exercising, there's always a risk of injury, no matter how careful you are. If you're training too frequently however, your muscles and joints are far more susceptible to injury.

If you are constantly putting your muscles, joints, and tendons under pressure when training, they will weaken and become more vulnerable.

Rest days, however, allow various parts of your body to recover and to become bigger and stronger once more. If you're looking to avoid injury rest and recovery days are extremely beneficial.

Improves athletic performance – If you're going to gym seven days a week, training for hours on end, you'll find yourself physically and mentally drained and burnt out.

And because you're so tired you won't be able to perform at your best. Taking a couple of rest and recovery days each week however, will help you to replenish your physical and mental energy so you get more done in the gym, or wherever else you choose to exercise.

Conclusion – Final Thoughts On Losing Weight Permanently

Congratulations on making it to the end of this short, introductory guide on losing weight easily, quickly and permanently.

As you now know, losing weight is not about following fad diets and making small changes here and there, it's about a total lifestyle overhaul.

There are no quick fixes when it comes to weight loss, but like anything in life, the more you know about it, the easier it becomes.

To help make your weight loss journey that little bit easier, we're now going to wrap things up by sharing a few tried and tested tips for losing weight and improving your fitness in a safe and controlled manner.

Start today – Have you ever noticed how people complaining about wanting to lose weight will always claim to be starting their diet and healthy eating regime on a Monday?

It could be a Wednesday and the individual wanting to lose weight would still claim to be starting their diet on a Monday. This is usually so that they can stuff their faces for the next several days as a final blow out, as they may call it, which means that they usually gain even more weight.

Stop looking for excuses, stop waiting until Monday, and instead, start your healthy eating and fitness regime t.o.d.a.y. The sooner you start and get off the mark, the sooner you will start seeing results.

Consider your long-term goals – Another thing you can do to ensure that you lose weight and stick to your healthy lifestyle is to consider long-term goals.

Don't just think about how much fat you want to lose, consider your long-term goals as well. Where do you want to be a year, two years, five years from now? Is your weight loss sustainable and are you willing to change your lifestyle instead of simply crash dieting and yo-yo dieting?

Change your lifestyle — If you're serious about getting in shape and staying in shape, it's essential that you change your lifestyle.

As mentioned, there is no quick fix for weight loss, and unfortunately, when most people lose weight quickly, they soon revert back to their old ways and gain the weight back, plus a little bit extra.

If you change your lifestyle however, that won't happen. You will learn healthy recipes and healthy habits that promote health and longevity, and help you to keep the weight off.

Have fun — Finally, if you are ready to commit to obtaining a leaner and healthier body, you need to make sure that you have fun and enjoy yourself. So many people out there follow diets that literally make them miserable, and then they wonder why they cheat or quit.

When you commit to getting in shape, try to have as much fun as you can. Eat healthy foods you enjoy, perform exercise you enjoy, and if you aren't enjoying yourself, look for things that you can do to turn that around.

Well thanks for joining me and continuing to the end. I wish you all the success in your future weight loss endeavors.

The Secret to Weight Loss for Life

If you missed it, the secret to weight loss for life is three-fold:

1. Eat healthy – learn the healthy nutritious foods to eat and in the right portions.
2. Exercise – Not only does it burn more calories, but it builds lean muscle mass which will increase your calorie burn in the future.
3. Live a healthy lifestyle – Ditch your unhealthy habits like smoking, abusing drugs or alcohol and focus instead on a healthy eating and exercising routine that you can live on for the rest of your life.

The links in this book are written by me and are there to give you additional sources of information about the highlighted topics that when learned can help you lose even more weight, get fit and healthy, and ultimately live longer!

About the Author

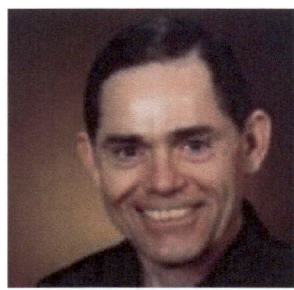

I have published numerous books on Amazon (both for Kindle and in paperback), along with other publishing platforms.

While most of my books are on health and fitness in general, I also write on baby boomer and older citizen health issues and have a recent interest in creating and printing journals/ planners and other printable products.

A complete list of our published products on Amazon can be found at https://www.amazon.com/Ron-Kness/e/B0072M6PYO.

Besides my own writing, I also ghostwrite ebooks, books, reports, articles, blogs and do Kindle conversions for clients on a variety of topics. Contact me at Ron Kness Writing for a quote.

Today my wife and I are retired from our careers and live in San Tan Valley, AZ. I now write as a retirement business where you'll find me happily sitting in my office typing away on my laptop as I work on my next book or ghostwriting project . . . that is if we are not traveling on a cruise ship - our new-found mode of travel.